Table of Contents

Preface

There was also a time when the study of losing weight did not indeed do in our society, people ate what mama cooked of r regale and they went to work. The difference in that society and moments so cite is that work wasn't behind a computer screen, but on their bases in the fields or on a storehouse bottom. People worked d physically because that was the only way to work, infect, that is why it was called work! It was hourly a during this time that people could eat anything they wanted because they were burning much further calories than what they consumed.

But, like all good effects, that too has passed and the technology of moment's world has left us in one condition – a fat bone. Our life styles have changed so drastically and our comforts have increased tenfold. As they say, every rose has its nuisance and for our society our desire to have comfortable lives and to work less has begun to show around the midriff.

The bad thing about all of this is the more weight you gain, the more dangerous it becomes. Redundant weight spells illness, whether it's in the form of diabetes or a heart condition, it's bound to show up if you do not do commodity about it. You have to be proactive in weight gain and you have to work it off until it gets to a point where you no longer have control. It's not inescapably about being toned and carved, but at a weight that isn't life hanging. You can work on the abs latterly, right now you just need to exfoliate some redundant body fat. As society realizes what's passing and that we're fat as a whole, people are trying to play catch over and work from behind. They're trying to lose weight and live a healthier life.

This eBook is your companion to losing that first ten pounds that we all struggle with. It's amazing what little changes in your life can add up to you losing ten pounds and they all revolve around eating right and getting your body moving.

Chapter 1

Weight loss Beginning with What You Drink

First and foremost, people do not realize that what they drink is the first step in losing that first 10 pounds. In fact, utmost people do not know that when they feel empty, they may actually be dehydrated and they're really thirsty, not empty. Water is remarkable as well. Over 66 of your body weight is nothing but water. This is also why water plays an important part in weight control. So, \

TIP# 1 is Drink plenitude of water. It's recommended that you drink 8 spectacles per day, but that may take you some time to work up to. Your body needs a whole lot of water. Water does not just flush all the to Xin's out of your body, but it makes you feel better and healthier. When you drink a lot of water you just begin to feel fit and this is the provocation you need to lose weight.

The stylish thing about water is you can drink as much as you want because it has no calories at all. When you are drinking a lot of water, you eat less as well because you will not feel as though you're starving to death. Remember, if you feel empty, try drinking a glass of water first and you will realize you were presumably just dehydrated and not empty at all.

The whole 8 spectacles a day rule is really something you should strive for. The stylish way to do this and to measure your water input is to buy a flagon from the medicine store or grocery store that's designed to hold exactly 8 spectacles of water. These are great weight loss tools because you can fill them up, indurate them and as it melts throughout the day you have fresh an d cold water. Or, if you do not mind your water room temperature you can drink it that way as well. All that matters is that you are getting in the water your body needs.

TIP# 2 Launch off your day with a fresh, clean glass of water. As soon as you get up in the morning, drink one down. This will help your body to get going because it will not be fighting through dehydration. Also, after you drink a glass of water you will not need to eat such a large breakfast. A glass of water wakes up all the digestive authorities in your body and gets it well lubricated. You can always have your morning coffee or tea, but be sure to have a glass of water latterly. Caffeine dehydrates you an d you want to shield off dehumidification.

TIP# 3 Drink a glass of water before you sit down to eat. Water will naturally make you feel fuller so you do not have to eat as important food.

TIP# 4 Have a glass of water while you eat as well. Take a drink after each bite and you'll feel full more snappily so you can leave the table feeling satisfied

without feeling bloated. Drinking water while you eat will also help your food to settle more snappily, which also helps you to feel full briskly.

TIP# 5 Do your stylish to stay down from so da. All tonics are candied with lots of sugar. The more you can cut out of your diet the better. Also, diet pop is still pop. It may not have as important sugar, but it has other chemicals and factors that aren't good for your body either. However, if you drink a pop. counteract it with a glass of water. Re member, caffeine dehydrates you as well. Decaffeinated tonics still have caffeine in small quantities as well and just as important sugar, so they aren't important healthier either.

TIP# 6 Fruit juice is not as healthy as utmost people suppose either. Juice actually has a lot of sugar in it as well. However, drink fresh fruit juice rather of juice that has artificial flavors and coloring, if you're pining a glass of juice. It's indeed better if you can make your own fruit juice. Just be sure not to add too important sugar which adds to the calories. Rather of drink fruit juice, eat more fruit. Fruit provides your body with important demanded fiber as well as vitamins.

TIP# 7 Go readily on the tea and coffee. They're enough much inoffensive if you do not add a lot of cream and sugar to t verge. It's the cream and sugar that becomes fattening. Suppose of it this way, when you have a mug of coffee or tea with cream and two cells of sugar, you are basically eating a piece of chocolate cake every time. Now suppose of how numerous pieces of cake you're eating when you have a Venti Starbucks Latte – yikes.

TIP# 8 If you must have your tea and coffee, try to drink it black. Black tea or coffee actually has health benefits to it as long as you counteract the caffeine in your body with a nice big glass of water. Caffeine is also not good for you because it affects functions in your body, like your metabolism.

Another type of tea that you can drink freely is green tea. Green tea has been used as a drug in China for over 0 times. It aids the digestive system and can help ease an exorbitantly full stoma ch and it has been linked to a reduction in cancer threat.

TIP# 9 If you can say no to alcohol, also that's stylish. Alcohol potables are not exactly good for you, although a glass of red wine does have heart benefits, utmost is just fattening. Beer is especially fattening. Amalgamations are fattening depending on what they're made of. For case, whiskey and Coke. The whiskey may not be fattening, but the Coke surely is. Plus, after a many drinks utmost people get the munchies and when you are feeling a little inebriated and empty you will not be suitable to make rational opinions regarding your diet and it's generally late at night, just before you pass out from a night of drinking, that you gormandize. The overall combination n is just not a good bone.

TIP# 10 If you must have alcohol, try dry wine. Dry wine is better than your sweet wines, because sweet wines have more sugar! Dry wines have sugar, but utmost of it has been instigated down in to alcohol and from a weight gaining perspective, dry is better.

TIP# 11 Another word on coffee, that isn't inescapably bad, but more intriguing than anything. Some people have reported that when they drank black coffee before exercising, they lost further weight. There is no scientific evidence to back this, but nutritionist s believe it may be caused by the body being forced to depend on fat for energy. Hey, it's worth trying if you can stage black coffee. Just remember to drink plenitude of water during your exercise!

TIP# 12 Avoid drinking inordinate quantities of coffee, as it desensitizes your body to the natural fat burning goods that c affine has. One or two mugs (if the days really slow to get started) maximum.

Chapter 2

Eating Well and Losing the Pounds

Okay, when utmost people suppose about losing weight and eating, they suppose about overeating. Well, unfortunately, all of the style diets out there tend to cause people to gain weight. Why? Because they starve them to death and the person ultimately breaks down and eats everything in sight because they're so infernal empty. They also deprive them of the foods that they love. This isn't a way to lose weight, nor is it a way to live. You only cause yourself stress, which actually causes you to gain weight!

So, in eating right there many tips that you can follow each and every day and they are not going to deprive you of the foods that you love, but treat those foods as luxury particulars so you enjoy them that much further.

TIP# 13 Eat fresh fruit and vegetables that have high water content. These are foods like tomatoes, watermelons, cantaloupe, kiwi, grapes – you get the idea. All of those fresh and scrumptious juicy fruits and veggies are good for you. These particulars contain about 90 to 95 waters, so you can eat a lot of these and they will fill you up without adding on the pounds.

TIP# 14 Eat fresh fruit rather of reused fruit. Anything that's reused as further sugar. Processed and c amend fruits also don't have as important fiber as fresh fruits.

TIP# 15 Increase your fiber input as much as you can. This generally means eating further fruits and veggies.

TIP# 16 Veggies are your musketeers when it comes to slipping pounds. There are tons of options then and you may indeed want to try some you have not had in the history. The lush green varieties are the stylish and you always want to work in a salad when you can. Salads are packed with nutrients as long as you do not pour too important dressing on and load them with too important rubbish. The lush flora also has a lot of natural water.

TIP# 17 Be intelligent about what you eat. Do not eat just to eat. Creatures eat on instinct; people eat when they know their body really needs it. Do not be an impulse eater.

TIP# 18 Watch everything you consume from the food itself to what you eclipse it with. Beautifiers and seasonings c a n sabotage a healthy mess because they are typic supporter high in fat.

TIP# 19 Get a handle on the sweet tooth. This does not mean you can't have your sweets; just do not eat them as a mess. Always remember that these sweets end up adding to an area that you do not want them to add to. Do not deprive yourself either however, because also you'll eat doubly as numerous as you should.

TIP# 20 Set mess times and stick to them. Try to have your reflections at specific times and eat them at that time. An eating pattern will help you to control what you eat and when you eat it. Also, it really is better to have 5 small reflections a day rather than just one or two huge reflections. Just eating once, a day makes your body feel as though it's starving, which packs on fat in vantage of using it as energy.

Also, do not stay until your starving to eat. This only makes you gormandize until you are stuffed.

TIP# 21 Eat only when you're empty. Be sure to drink a glass of water first to determine if you really are empty or if you are really thirsty. Numerous people have the tendency to eat when they see food. It does not mean they're empty; they just want to eat it. Do not eat anything you are offered unless you really are, just mouthful, do not have a mess, if you feel you must eat it out of being polite.

TIP# 22 Try not to snack between reflections, but if you must have a snack make sure it's a healthy bone. If you travel a lot, try to find healthy snacks and not junk food.

TIP# 23 Veggies make great snacks. They can get you through the hunger stings if you're having t verge. Carrots are great because they satisfy hunger and they're dad caked with nutrients.

TIP# 24 Counting calories is a good idea for those must have food items. However, also it'll have the calories on the dad caking, if it's a dad caked food item. Be sure to pay attention to serving sizes in terms of calories as well. An Otis Spunkmeyer muffin is intended to be two servings, so you have to double the calories listed. This is where food directors get tricky and you can't fall in their trap.

TIP# 25 Work off the redundant calories by the end of the week. However, be sure to get to the spa or go walking a little If you feel you have splurged too important this week. longer to work off those redundant calories you have consumed.

TIP# 26 Stay down from all effects fried. However, it's better that it is If it's breaded. Baked. Fried foods are immersed in fat and canvas. Indeed, after the excess has canvas has been drained down, there's still canvas absorbed into the food item itself.

TIP# 27 Do not skip reflections. You should have, at the veritably least, three reflections a day, but rather five small reflections. This will keep you from getting empty during the day and gorging out of starvation.

TIP# 28 Just like fruits, fresh vegetables are better than those that are canned. It's indeed better if you can eat your veggies raw. When you cook them, you cook down the nutrients? However, try to boil them to the point If you must co othermother there's still some crisp ness to them. Also, do not soak them in butter. However, that's indeed better, If you can steal organic and fungicide free veggies.

TIP# 29 Do not eat further than one egg per day. It's stylish if you can reduce your egg input to three a week.

TIP# 30 Chocolates should be treated as luxury particulars. Buy the good stuff and only eat them every formerly in a while. However, you'll If you really savor each morsel. experience that much further joy in eating them and they will taste indeed better.

TIP# 31 Eat foods from all of the food groups each day. This is a great way to insure you're getting all the nutrients your body needs and it helps to shield off any diet scarcities. Also, do not eat the same foods all the time. Trial so that you do not get wearied with same old diet.

TIP# 32 Try to eat breakfast within an hour of waking up. This is the stylish way to give your body the jump start it needs. Do not stay until you're really empty. Breakfast is important, but you do not need to stuff yourself. The idea is that you are breaking the fast from not easting all night.

TIP# 33 Your diet should include all aspects of the food groups including carbohydrates. In fact, your diet needs to be about 50-55 c arbs. Carbs are a great source of energy. Those diets that enjoin carbohydrates are actually harming you and only making you crave them that much further. Your diet should cause you to be deficient in anything.

TIP# 34 Proteins should make up only 25-30 of your diet. Far too important emphasis is put on meat as the main part of your mess. In actuality, it should bucconid erred further of a side dish rather than the main course.

TIP# 35 Fats should make up 15-20 of your meal. This is really all the fat your body needs. A lot of this is going to be in your diet in the form of cream, sugar and the suchlike.

TIP# 36 Eat further white meat than red meat. White meat includes funk, fish and some other fowl. Red meat includes beef and pork.

TIP# 37 Try to go as submissive as you can. This really is a healthier life, indeed if you can't cut meat out fully. The further fruits and veggies you can eat the better. The further meat you cut out, the more fat you can cut out of your diet as well. Still, protein is important, so be certain that your option allows you to maintain good protein situations.

TIP# 38 White chuck is good, but high fiber multigrain viands are much better. These viands are another way to add further fiber to your diet and they also have a good protein position.

TIP# 39 Pork doesn't help in weight loss in any way. The less pork you eat, the better off you'll be when trying to lose weight. Pork has a high fat content and includes food particulars similar as ba con, ham and link.

TIP# 40 Limit your sugar input as much as possible. However, try to find an artificial sweetener that you do not mind the taste of, if you must have sweetener in your coffee and tea. Still, these things aren't all that healthy either and should be limited as well.

TIP# 41 Try grazing five to six times a day. These are those small reflections we bandied before. Some people lose weight more when they no way feel empty and grazing on healthy food particulars can do this for you. Plus, it keeps your metabolism working, which will burn fat naturally.

TIP# 42 Do not worry about cheating, but don't cheat for a mess. Eat sweets and your favorite cheat food for the flavor only. However, share one with the whole family, If you want cate after regale. You will get the flavor, but not the pounds.

TIP# 43 Watch your fat input. Each fat gram is 9 calories. If you know your total calories also you can figure the quantum of fat in those particulars.

TIP# 44 Take it easy on the swab and try to cu t what you use in half. Swab is one of the main causes of rotundity.

Chapter 3

Lose weight By Changing How You Cook

Then are many tips that will help you to lose those first ten pounds by simply changing how you prepare your food. How food is cooked has just as important to do with how healthy it's or is not.

TIP# 45 Rather of frying in canvas or fat, try baking those particulars isn't ead. Baking doesn't bear all the fat and canvas that frying requires and your food isn't soaking in those substances while its culinarians.

TIP# 46 Use on-stick frying visage spray so you do not use canvas. Also, kissers that arenol-stick do not bear as much, if any canvas.

TIP# 47 Pustule vegetables rather of cooking them. You can also foam them, as this is presumably the healthiest way to eat foods like cabbages, cauliflower, broccoli and carrots.

TIP# 48 Be leery of no fat and low-fat food particulars. There are numerous of these food particulars on the request, but they aren't exactly healthy. Numerous of these food particulars use some kind of chemical or carbohydrate to candy them so that they taste better. Still, the body turns these chemicals and carbohydrates into sugar in the body, which means they're still getting turned into fat.

TIP# 49 Do not fall victim to crash diets. These are bad for you and do more detriment than good in the long run. The short-term results are typic supporter that you'll lose a many pounds, but once you give them up also everything comes back and your weight is worse the alternate time around. You cannot survive on a crash diet and you ultimately get to a po int where you have to give it up.

TIP# 50 Bite your food at least 8 to 12 times whether it's liquid food, sweets or ice cream. This adds slaver to the food that digests the sugar. When food isn't eaten duly and is just swallowed, you fill your stomach with food that is not ready to be digested and it also doesn't yield the health benefits that you need.

TIP# 51 When you're cooking with canvas, use a good Extra Virgin Olive Oil. It is more precious than vegetable canvas, but the health benefits are much better and it's worth the cost. Olive canvas has been associated with a reduced threat in coronary heart complaint and helps to increase the plainness of the arterial walls which reduces the chance for heart atta ck and stroke.

Chapter 4

Exercising To Lose Weight

There are two effects that you must do to lose weight and one of those we've formerly covered enough considerably and that's to eat right and fill your body with good, clean water. The other thing you have to do is get your body moving. You do not have to buy a spa class to get exercise. Infect, there are several affects you can do on a diurnal base that will help to protest start your body into losing weight and there are several exercises you can do on your own to lose weight.

TIP# 52 When you begin working out, whether at home or in a spa, do not be discouraged if you do not see results right down. It takes further than a week to get your body into shape and to begin maki ng progress. Numerous people make the mistake of believing that their exercising is not working when it just takes a little bit of time.

If you push your body too important when you first get started exercising you can end up with injuries. Your bones, joints and ligaments aren't prepared for the exertion you're putting on them. Do not suppose that if you really push yourself hard for many exercises that you will lose plutocrat, unfortunately the body does not work this way. Slow and steady wins the race when it comes to exercising.

TIP# 53 Check your weight when you start exercising, but do not us e it as a companion to how important weight you're losing. Your weight fluctuates throughout the day. Still, you may only end up getting discouraged, If you check your weight every day.

TIP# 54 The stylish way to know if you are losing weight is by the fit of your clothes. If you start to feel as though you are floating in your clothes also you know you are eating and exercising is doing you some good. Another way to know if you are losing weight is if you can begin moving where you generally buckle your belt, of course tighter is better.

TIP# 55 When your periodic supporter checks your weight and the fit of your clothes, award yourself. Buy yourself some new handling shoes or a new brace of jeans. This will help to keep you motivated as you pursue your weight loss pretensions.

TIP# 56 Take a day off from exercising to give your body with a chance to rest and repair. Your body needs a day out formerly a week.

TIP# 57 Three days of 30 nanosecond exercise will help you to maintain your weight, but you need at least 4 days of 30 nanosecond exercise to begin to lose weight and 5 days a week is indeed better.

TIP# 58 Collect information on exercise and easy affects you can do from your own home. There're tons of expansive exploration available on exercise and you can choose what will help you the most to meet your weight loss pretensions. Browse the Internet or pick up some books on health and exercise from your loc al bookstore or library to learn further and how to burn off the desire d number of calories you're trying to burn each week.

TIP# 59 Try to find an exercise chum. This should be someone who's as married to exercising and losing weight as you are. One of the advantages of chancing a married mate is that you have someone to keep feeling responsible to them. The knowledge that someone is staying on you makes it easier for you to get out of bed and go exercise with them. You wouldn't want to stand up your exercise chum, would you?

TIP# 60 When your body tells you it has had enough, take a break. When you have worked out for a considerable amount of time, you'll start entering signals from your body. This is particularly important when you're just getting started in your exercise routine.

TIP# 61 If you decide to increase the length of your exercises, do so gradationally. The same is true for the intensity of your exercises.

TIP# 62 Elect an exercise routine that suits your life. Everybody has a different life and a different profession. There's no set time that you should or shouldn't drill. If you like to drill late before you go to bed because it's relaxing to you also, do it. If you like to drill beforehand in the morning because it helps you wake up also that is great too. Some people like to drill on their lunch break to take a break from the stress of their job or because that's the only time they've available.

TIP# 63 Do not stand around, walk around. If you can walk around also, do it. People who are dancers are actually doing themselves a lot of good because they're constantly moving. Pacing also helps you suppose.

TIP# 64 Do not sit if you can stand. However, you'll burn further calories doing so than if you were to sit, if you can stage comfortably.

TIP# 65 Do not lie down if you can sit. Same conception as the two over.

TIP# 66 The settee and the TV areanti-weightloss. However, do not sit on it, If you're inclined to come a settee potato. In fact, if you have to, put a not so comfortable president in front of the TV so you will not spend so important time in front of it. The same is true for the presentation utter if you are a computer junkie. Some people have a more comfortable president in front of their computer than they do in front of their TV. (This is, of course, if you do not work from home and need to work hours at a time in front of your computer because your president is veritably important also.)

TIP# 67 If you have a job where you sit the whole time, stand up and stretch every partial hour or so. Utmost of moment's jobs are in front of a computer and bear you to sit. If you have a job like this, make it a point to move every so frequently.

TIP# 68 Walk around while you are on the telephone. You will get a good drill if it's a long discussion.

TIP# 69 Use the stairs rather of the elevator or escalator. These are great conveniences, but they make us veritably lazy. Also, it may be hastily to take the stairs than to stay on an elevator to open.

TIP# 70 Quit smoking. Smoking doesn't cont. tribute to your weight exa ctly, but it does lead to era tic eating behaviors and increases caffeine dependence.

TIP# 71 10 twinkles of cardio a day is good for utmost, you can get this by other styles than running.

TIP# 72 If you can't run for a physical reason, also try 15 twinkles of brisk walking to keep fit.

TIP# 73 You can walk anywhere if you have time. However, consider walking there or riding-riding-doing a bike, If work or the grocery store isn't far down. It may take you longer,

but you are getting your drill in at the same time.

TIP# 74 Hide the remote control from yourself. Remote controls are also evil when it comes to losing weight. However, you may not indeed turn on the TV, which means you might find more active effects to do, if you did not have a remote. Get up and change the channel if you do not have a remote or go for a walk rather of watching Television.

TIP# 75 Do your own fetching. However, the Television channel changed, the correspondence or review from the driveway, if you need commodity from the kitchen. Adding a little walking to your day will do prodigies for you.

TIP# 76 Walk along or climb the escalator with it or just take the stairs.

TIP# 77 Walk around during marketable breaks or do simple exercises like crunches or bending over and touching your toes. Do anything to get your body moving more and to keep your blood pumping.

TIP# 78 Turn on some music and cotillion. Again, the more you get moving the better you'll feel and the further weight you'll lose.

TIP# 79 If you take public transportation, get off a block before your stop and walk the remainder of the way. This is a good way to squeeze in a walk ahead and after work or on the way to another destination.

TIP# 80 Do pelvic rotations to get your midsection in shape. Of course, you wouldn't do these with anybody around, but they're a good step in getting your body prepared for more serious stomach crunches. It's also good on the back muscles and keeps you lose rather of tight.

TIP# 81 Stink in your stomach when you walk. Walk duly, but do your stylish to keep that stomach partake in. You'll soon begin to feel those muscles tightening.

TIP# 82 Do breathe exercises to tone your waist. It's amazing how breathing duly and with your entire diaphragm can actually help to strain your abdominal muscles. Utmost people breathe way too shallow as it's an oxygen is good for the brain.

TIP# 83 Trial with yoga. Yoga is a great way to lose weight and reduce your stress situations. Yoga teaches you how to control your muscles and gain further control of your individual muscle's groups.

TIP# 84 Lift weights. Strength training burns more fat than people give it credit. When you work on structure muscle, they begin to burn fat to fuel muscles growth. Do be apprehensive that when you ga in muscle, your scale may not be an accurate tool in determining weight loss because muscle weighs further than fat.

TIP# 85 Massage your mate. You can exert yourself a little bit and at the same time you'll be suitable to round them on the weight they've lost if they've been working out with you.

TIP# 86 Take the stairs two at a time rather of one at a time. This causes you to have to ply yourself more and increases your heart rate.

TIP# 87 Take your canine on a walk. Chance s are that if you are not getting enough exercise, neither is your pet. Or, let your canine take you on a walk. For formerly in his life, let him lead you where he wants to go and as presto as he wants to get there. It could be a good drill for the both of you.

TIP# 88 Join a dancing class. This could be chamber dancing where you learn balls like the tango, salsa or fox witch. These balls are fast dad cede and will get you moving. Indeed, slow chamber dancing is a lot of exercise and will surely tone your legs. Or, you can take an aerobic cotillion class. How numerous hops do you know that are fat?

TIP# 89 Spare against the wall so that your face is close and also use your hands to push your body down. Do these three or four times to stretch.

TIP# 90 Syncope whenever you can. Swimming is a great way to get your c ardio exercise and it's low to no impact on your joints, which is great for people who have osteoporosis or joint problems.

TIP# 91 Try playing tennis or handbasket ball. Playing games are a great way to get into shape. It's also further fun to wo rkout with someone differently in a competitive atmosphere. You'll be more driven to push yourself and you will burn further calories, just do not overstate it.

TIP# 92 Always start your drill with a warm up of about 5-10 twinkles and end with a cool down of 5-10 twinkles. Your body needs to rea ch a certain heart rate position before it'll respond well to the rest of the drill.

TIP# 93 Do not carry your wireless phone or cell phone withyou. However, go walk for it, if it rings. There are so numerous convene inches in life and we always have everything we need at our fingertips, but this is obviously bad for the midriff.

TIP# 94 If you are standing around, stretch your legs a bit by standing up on your toes and also gradationally drop to you heals. You can also flex your buttock muscles as well, but perhaps when nothing differently is looking.

TIP# 95 Before going to bed, undress and gawk at yourself in front of the glass. Take note of what areas you need to ameliorate on and what areas are your stylish means. Taking a tone- force can keep you motivated in your drill trials. Also, do not forget to compel meant yourself on any new muscle tone you may have or other advancements you've made.

TIP# 96 Do not slouch in your president. Try to sit up straight and erect at all times. Limping is bad for your back and gives you a squooshy figure. Make it a point to always sit and stand with good posture.

TIP# 97 Utmost people would like to target their stomachs and get relieve of that area each together. Unfortunately, we can't spot reduce. But, one thing you can do is a breathing exercise to help strain those stomach muscles. Breathe in air as strong as you can and tuck your stomach at the same time as much as you can. Hold it for a many alternate s and also sluggishly let it out. Do not let it out so presto that your belly flops out. This isn't good. Try to breathe like this whenever you suppose about it, about 50–60-time s a day is ideal. This will help you to lose at least an inch within 20 days or so.

TIP# 98 Use a map, similar as the one below to help you in your weight loss trials. This map shows you how numerous calories each of these common exercises burn, grounded on 20 twinkles.

Exercise	Calories Burned
Calisthenics	200-250
Stationary Bicycling	250-300
Factual Bicycling	300-400
Handling at 5-6 mph	300-350
Stair climber	200-250
Swimming Laps	350
Brisk Walking	150-180
Weeding and Cultivating Your Garden	130-200
Coitus (Yes, coitus can be exercise too)	50-60

Basketball – firing baskets to playing a game	130-250
Golf – carrying clubs, no c art	166
Golf – carrying clubs, grounded on 2 hours of play rather of 20 twinkles	1000
Snorkeling	150-200
Water Skiing	180-200
Ice Skating – general	200-250
Cross Country Skiing,2.5 mph, light trouble	200-250
General Skiing	200-250
Scuba Diving	200-250
Chute rafting, kayaking or canoeing	150-200
Flag or Touch Football	250-300
Horseback Riding – Sprinting	200-250
Martial Trades	300-350
Ra cquetball	200-250
Volleyball – 6-to-9-person platoon	90-120
Volleyball – Beach	25-300
Tennis – mates	250-300
Tai Chi	120-180

* Your results will depend on how important you presently weigh as well. If you're looking for an accurate calculation grounded on your body weight and details of the exercise you're performing go toiVillage.com at

From this map you can see that walking is a great way to get exercise. However, a good walk is a good launch, If you are too busy to do any of the other exercises.

TIP# 99 Do not discourage yourself from exercising and eating right by wearing clothes that donutty. However, wear a medium, if you are a medium. Wearing the wrong types of clothes can make you appear larger than you really are. This includes drill wear as well. However, you get to go shopping latterly for lower clothes and you can send your slightly worn larger clothes in a

If you wear clothes that fit now. consignment shop or you can take them to Goodwill to be given to someone who can use them.

Chapter 5

Getting Started

Now that you understand how to get started, then is a little further information on losing weight and keeping it off and it all begins with what you eat.

Fat and weight loss is such an important aspect in our life moment because we're fatter now than we've ever been. Th e word" weight loss programs "will catch the attention of anybody harkening in on a discussion or watching TV. Infect, that is one of the most popular keywords searched on the Internet moment.

The main reason that we're sovereign hit is because of our relationship with food. In our society, we tend to connect rate on volume. We sim ply want as important as we can get rather of the stylish food that we can progeny. Volume always beats out quality, when it should be exactly the contrary of that.

Once you've decided to lose weight, it can be delicate to determine where exactly you should get started. However, it's possible, if you have a strong resoluteness to get going and to lose weight. You just have to figure out how to say "no."

Everybody is different. You are not going to find another person who has the same metabolism as you or who burns fat the same way as you. You may weigh exactly the same as a person coming to you, but if you both were to start an exercise and diet program you both might not have the same results two weeks or indeed a month latterly, indeed if you did everything the same exact way each day. In saying this, it's important to realize that not everybody utilizes food in the same way moreover. What may cause one person to gain a pound may not do the same to another. The same is true in lo sing weight. If you are a wedded woman and you and your hubby are working out together and let's, say he gives up pop and loses five pounds from stopping his input of pop and you do not lose

one pound, that shows you that you and your hubby aren't inescapably going to see the same results, indeed if you're eating and exercising in the exact same way.

The nethermost line is that moment's society has to work a lot harder than societies of the history. Sixty times ago women and men were thin because they had to work. Homemade labor was a demand or you wouldn't be suitable to eat. You had to go gather eggs from the hen house if you want eggs, you had to go milk the cows for fresh milk and you had to plow the fi elds to grow your vegetables. If you wanted beef, well you had to know a little commodity about fattening up a c alf and getting it butchered. That is the way life was back also and technology has taken down all of this homemade work. So, rather we've to watch what we eat and we've to go make ourselves exercise. If we do not, we do not have a reason to move half the time.

It's veritably important to understand that you weight loss pretensions are veritably dependent on how much you're willing to work at it. It's the one thing in life that you have to do homemade labor to a chive if you want to see results.

Generally, people don't need to worry about weight loss until their twenties, but with the fast-food life that we live moment this isn't inescapably the case presently. Numerous of our children are fat because they eat too important fast food and reused foods. When you are grocery shopping for yourself and your family read the constituents of what you're eating. However, do not eat it, if you can't gasp it. Reused foods cause to have jones and jones cause us to gain weight. This is particularly important to understand if you're ever going to be effective at losing weight and keeping it off.

Watching your diet alone isn't going to make you lose weight however. The proper diet has to be paired with the proper quantum of exercise as well. The result is an exercise troop that will give your body the exercise it needs to burn fat and c aloriesefficiently. However, it's like you are in hibernation and your body just dad cos on the pounds, particularly around your midriff, if you don't move.

Working Out Really Is Good for You

When you suppose about life in the once when your sweat was caused by hard work and the sun, it just makes you feel good each over. The sun beating down on your shoulders and the strain on your muscles just makes you feel stronger all over.

There really is nothing better than working out – outside.

But utmost people have moved to the megacity. The days of working on the ranch are long gone for utmost, still, there are a many people who still get to have that noble feeling of doing work and producing commodity that was real and keep the pounds off while they do it. Seriously, if you suppose about it, how numerous ranch hands, cowhands and drovers are fat? There are not numerous. Suppose about their cultures. They get up, have a mug of coffee and breakfast, go to work, come in for lunch, go to work, come in for regale and also go to bed beforehand enough to get up in the morning and do it each over again. In the meantime, they get good sun and fresh air and consume fresh water all day long. It truly is a healthy life. Unfortunately, utmost of us works outdoors, sitting down and still eat three reflections a day but have to do it so snappily you do not indeed get the occasion to taste it.

It's a fact of life that people in the megacity do not get important exercise, unless you live in a megacity where you walk everyplace you go. This means you have to put your mind to it and work at it. You have to fi t fitness into your diurnal schedule or you are going to be fat and sick. That is just the way it is. Exercise is the stylish way to control rotundity, it's the stylish way to control stress, hypertension, cardio vascular complaint, and other life relate dillnesses. However, indeed more, If you can drill outdoors. Your body needs as important fresh air as it can progeny.

Thickness

Thickness is the most important aspect of any exercise program. However, also if you constantly work towards that thing, you will be suitable to reach it, if you have a thing.

Getting started is generally easy for people. They go shopping, get some drill clothes, buy some handling shoes and perhaps a spa class. Also, they go and drill enough steadily for a week or two.

But, as they go, they find it harder to keep up their routine. Their lives come more demanding and they begin to go to the spa less and less. In other words, their spa class goes to west e and they just stop going.

Numerous people choose to drill in the evenings, but for some this routine is indeed harder to keep going. However, also this is a good time to go, if you are not fully exhausted when you get off from work. But, if you cannot also you may need to find a way to get there in the morning. It'll help you to get woke up and you will be suitable to maintain your consistency.

There's a misconception that exercise makes you tired, but that is not inescapably the case. It may do this to you the first many times, but as you get fit, you'll find you have further energy. Couple exercise with acceptable sleep, you shouldn't have any problem getting up in the morning and getting going. Plus, you will be amped all day long, which will help you to make it through your workday much easier.

Indeed, if you do not have a gym class, chances are that there's a side walk outside your house and some people ma y indeed have access to a pool. Get up a partial hour before, throw on the lurkers and get to walking, running, jogging or whatever your exercise of choices. However, they'll surely enjoy this time with you as well, If you have a four lawful friend.

www.ingramcontent.com/pod-product-compliance
Lightning Source LLC
LaVergne TN
LVHW080600160826
845677LV00010B/1932
9798846032385